Laura Verónica Partida Jasso
Manuel Arturo Rivas González

Risk factors for CKD in patients with Type 2 Diabetes Mellitus

Laura Verónica Partida Jasso
Manuel Arturo Rivas González

Risk factors for CKD in patients with Type 2 Diabetes Mellitus

Occurrence and progression of chronic kidney disease in patients with diabetes mellitus

ScienciaScripts

Imprint
Any brand names and product names mentioned in this book are subject to trademark, brand or patent protection and are trademarks or registered trademarks of their respective holders. The use of brand names, product names, common names, trade names, product descriptions etc. even without a particular marking in this work is in no way to be construed to mean that such names may be regarded as unrestricted in respect of trademark and brand protection legislation and could thus be used by anyone.

Cover image: www.ingimage.com

This book is a translation from the original published under ISBN 978-620-0-01767-3.

Publisher:
Sciencia Scripts
is a trademark of
Dodo Books Indian Ocean Ltd. and OmniScriptum S.R.L publishing group

120 High Road, East Finchley, London, N2 9ED, United Kingdom
Str. Armeneasca 28/1, office 1, Chisinau MD-2012, Republic of Moldova, Europe
Managing Directors: Ieva Konstantinova, Victoria Ursu
info@omniscriptum.com

Printed at: see last page
ISBN: 978-620-8-61706-6

Contents

FOREWORD

This work is the result of scientific research conducted at clinic #49 of the Mexican Social Security Institute, located in the city of Victoria Durango, Durango, Mexico. The authors collected data from a sample of records of patients with diabetes mellitus 2 (DM2), in which emphasis was placed on those risk factors for developing Chronic Kidney Disease (CKD), in order to determine the frequency of these risk factors in patients with DM2. In this book the reader will find relevant information on the physiological disorders that commonly occur in people with DM2 and which of them lead to the development of CKD, as well as less common factors that need to be addressed to inhibit, as far as possible, the onset and progression of CKD. The risk factors for developing CKD considered in this study were: gender, nutritional status, age, hypertension, poorly controlled diabetes, nephrotoxic drugs, autoimmune diseases, poorly controlled hypertension, smoking, dyslipidaemia and anaemia. In the results and discussion section, the reader will find detailed information on the intensity and incidence of each risk factor studied, and in a more summarised form in the summary and conclusions. The information contained in all sections of this work is important for researchers, teachers, students, nursing staff, management, administrative staff, families and patients with the diseases mentioned.

Dr. Laura Verónica Partida Jasso

Dr. Manuel Arturo Rivas González

RISK FACTORS FOR THE OCCURRENCE AND PROGRESSION OF CHRONIC KIDNEY DISEASE (CKD) IN PATIENTS WITH TYPE 2 DIABETES

Diabetes Mellitus 2 (DM2) is a disease that is currently occurring very frequently in Mexican citizens, although it is also a problem worldwide, with individuals at risk of developing Chronic Kidney Disease (CKD) due to factors such as gender, nutritional status, age, high blood pressure, poorly controlled diabetes and nephrotoxic drugs; However, other factors such as autoimmune diseases, poorly controlled hypertension, smoking, dyslipidaemia and anaemia are also often present and, although less common in populations, also require attention in order to reduce them in populations with DM2 and, consequently, prevent or limit the onset and progression of CKD.

SUMMARY

This research was conducted at the UMF No. 49 of the IMSS in Ciudad Victoria Durango, Durango, with the aim of identifying the main risk factors for the onset and progression of CKD in patients with DM2. Information was collected from the records of 139 patients (men and women), making it possible to gather data on sex, weight, height, age, arterial hypertension, autoimmune diseases, nephrotoxic drugs, poorly controlled hypertension, poorly controlled diabetes, dyslipidaemia, smoking and anaemia, in order to resolve the question of which are the risk factors for the onset and progression of CKD in patients with DM2 in the UMF No 49, by taking into account the frequency of each of the variables mentioned. The results indicated that the main risk factors for the onset and progression of CKD in patients with DM2 in UMF No. 49 were gender, nutritional status, age, hypertension, poorly controlled diabetes and nephrotoxic drugs; while factors such as autoimmune diseases, poorly controlled hypertension, smoking, dyslipidaemia and anaemia were not very frequent in the population used for the research. However, they also require attention in order to reduce them further in the population with DM2 and CKD treated at UMF No. 49.

Keywords: Hypertension, poorly controlled diabetes, poorly controlled hypertension, nephrotoxic drugs, kidney damage.

I INTRODUCTION

Diabetes is a serious disease that occurs when the pancreas does not produce enough insulin or when the body cannot use the insulin it produces. This hormone controls the amount of glucose in the blood. High blood glucose can cause many problems in the body. Glucose comes from the food that is consumed by humans, and insulin is the hormone that helps this sugar enter the cells to provide them with the required energy (1).

There are two main types of diabetes mellitus, type 1 and type 2; the former is characterised by the body not producing insulin, while the latter is where the pancreas produces insulin but the body cannot use it properly. Pre diabetes, where the blood glucose level is elevated, but not high enough to be considered type 2 diabetes mellitus, is also known. There is also gestational diabetes mellitus, which refers to high blood glucose levels that cause problems in pregnant women (2).

Diabetes is one of the conditions that cause kidney damage, which in turn leads to people suffering from chronic kidney disease (CKD), which affects a high percentage of the population. CKD is also related to pathological conditions such as ageing, high blood pressure (HBP) and cardiovascular disease (3). It is therefore important to identify potential risk factors in patients with non-communicable diseases in a timely manner to minimise the likelihood of developing CKD (4).

It is clear and explained that CKD results from alterations in the structure and function of the kidneys. Based on the glomerular filtration rate (GFR), different stages of CKD have been established, which are: stage 1, when patients have kidney damage, e.g. protein in the urine, with normal GFR (>90); stage 2, patients with kidney damage and mildly decreased GFR (60-89); stage 3, subdivided depending on GFR (G3a 45-59 and G3b 30- 44); stage 4, patients with severely reduced GFR (15-29) and stage 5, patients with kidney failure with GFR <15 (3).

II THEORETICAL FRAMEWORK

2.1 Diabetes Mellitus

Diabetes Mellitus (diabetes) is a metabolic disorder with heterogeneous pathologies, characterised by chronic hyperglycaemia and disturbances of carbohydrate, fat and protein metabolism, resulting from defects in insulin secretion, insulin action or both (5).

Several pathogenic processes are involved in the development of diabetes. These include those that impair pancreatic beta cells and gradually impair their function and consequently lead to insulin deficiency or resistance to insulin action (insulin resistance/insulin insensitivity (6).

2.2 Classification of diabetes

- Type 1 diabetes mellitus (DM1) is usually diagnosed at an early age and is caused by autoimmune β-cell destruction, resulting in insulin deficiency (7).
- Type 2 Diabetes Mellitus (DM2) caused by a progressive loss of adequate β-cell insulin secretion, often in association with insulin resistance, which is mainly linked to sedentary and overweight individuals (7).
- Gestational diabetes mellitus, diagnosed during the second or third trimester of pregnancy, which is not obviously pre-gestational (7).
- Other types of diabetes due to other causes: e.g. monogenic diabetes syndrome, diseases of the exocrine pancreas (such as pancreatitis) and drug- or chemical-induced diabetes (glucocorticoid use, HIV/AIDS treatment, after organ transplantation) (7).

2.3 Diagnostic criteria

There are different ways to diagnose diabetes, such as tests that determine the level of glucose in the blood or the presence of classic symptoms of high blood glucose.

Table 1. ADA criteria for the diagnosis of diabetes.

Fasting glucose> 126 mg/dL (no caloric intake in the last 8 hours).

2-hour plasma glucose >200 mg/dL during an oral glucose tolerance test. The test should be performed with a 75 gram glucose load dissolved in water.

Glycosylated haemoglobin (HbA1C) > 6.5%.

Patient with classic symptoms of hyperglycaemia or hyperglycaemic crisis with a random glucose > 200 mg/dL.(3)

*ADA 2023.

2.4 Pathophysiology

According to the World Health Organisation (WHO), diabetes mellitus is a chronic metabolic disease characterised by high blood glucose levels, which over time leads to damage to the heart, vasculature, eyes, kidneys and nerves (8). More than 90% of diabetes mellitus cases are DM2, a condition characterised by impaired insulin secretion by the β-cells of the pancreatic islets, tissue insulin resistance (IR) and an inadequate compensatory insulin secretory response. Disease progression renders insulin secretion unable to maintain glucose homeostasis, resulting in hyperglycaemia. Patients with type 2 diabetes mellitus are mostly characterised by obesity or a higher percentage of body fat, predominantly distributed in the abdominal region. In this condition, adipose tissue promotes insulin resistance through several inflammatory mechanisms, including increased release of free fatty acids and dysregulation of adipokines. The main drivers of DM2 are the global increase in obesity, sedentary lifestyles, high-calorie diets and an ageing population, which have quadrupled the incidence and prevalence of DM2 (9).

Organs involved in the development of type 2 diabetes mellitus include the pancreas (β-cells and α-cells), liver, skeletal muscle, kidneys, brain, small intestine and adipose tissue. Evolving data suggest that adipokine dysregulation, inflammation and abnormalities in the gut microbiota, immune dysregulation and inflammation have emerged as important pathophysiological factors (9).

2.5 Epidemiology

Epidemiological data show alarming values that predict a worrying future for DM2. According to the International Diabetes Federation (IDF), in 2019, diabetes caused 4.2 million deaths; and 463 million adults aged 20-79 years were living with diabetes, a number that is likely to increase to 700 million by 2045. Diabetes was the underlying cause of at least $720 billion in healthcare spending in 2019. Furthermore, the disease burden of DM2 is likely to be under-represented, as saying one in three people with diabetes is perhaps an under-diagnosis, but it equates to 232 million people. The largest number of people with diabetes are aged 40-59 years. The incidence and prevalence of DM2 varies by geographic region, with more than 80% of patients living in low- to middle-income countries, posing additional challenges to effective treatment. Patients with DM2 have a 15% higher risk of all-cause mortality compared to people without diabetes, and cardiovascular disease (CVD) is the leading cause of morbidity and mortality associated with DM2. The association of diabetes with a increased risk of coronary heart disease, ischaemic stroke and other vascular disease-related deaths was shown in a meta-analysis (10).

2.6 Treatment

The treatment of DM2 should follow a sequence, devised by international consensus, which has placed emphasis on starting by modifying lifestyle according to diet and physical activity. The dietary regime focuses on providing the diabetic patient with sufficient macro- and micronutrients to preserve a normal weight and prevent glycaemia alterations. It is known that physical exercise allows glucose transport at the cell membrane level by a mechanism independent of insulin. If these measures are not suitable, treatment with oral hypoglycaemic agents should be initiated, either in monotherapy or in combination therapy, a list of drugs is given in table 2 (11).

Table 2. Group of oral antidiabetics.

Group	Drugs	Mechanism of action	HbA1c reduction	Effects on weight
Biguanides	Metformin	Decreases insulin resistance Stimulation of insulin secretion	High	Neutral/ decreases
Sulphonylureas	Glibenclamide Glipizide Glimepiride	Stimulation of insulin secretion.	High	Increase
Glinidas	Nateglitida Repaglinide	Stimulation of insulin secretion.	High	Neutral / loss
Thiazolidinediones	Pioglitazone Rosiglitazone	Increases insulin sensitivity and inhibition of hepatic glucose production.	High	Neutral / loss
α-Glucosidase inhibitors	Acarbose MIglitol	Reduced intestinal absorption of carbohydrates	Intermediate	Neutral
GLP1 agonists	Exenatide Liraglutide Albiglutide Dulaglutide	Stimulation of insulin secretion. Decreased glucagon. Delayed gastric emptying. Satiety	High	Loss
DPP-4 inhibitors	Sitagliptin Vidagliptin Saxagliptin Saxagliptin Linagliptin	Stimulation of insulin secretion. Decrease in glucagon.	Intermediate	Neutral
ISGLT2	Canaglizofine Daglizofine Empaglizofine	Glucosuria due to inhibition of renal reabsorption of glucose	Intermediate	Loss

Garmendia-Lorena **F. El tratamiento actual de la Diabetes Mellitus tipo 2. Diagnóstico (Lima). 2020;59(1):3-4**

2.7 Complications and risk factors

There are two broad groups of likely complications of diabetes: acute and chronic. Acute complications are hypoglycaemias and hyperglycaemias, while chronic complications are related to cardiovascular disease, retinopathies, nephropathies, cerebrovascular involvement that can lead to neuropathies, complications in the skin, mouth and the diabetic foot (2).

Risk factors for developing DM2 are related to genetic factors and unfavourable lifestyles, so specifically look at factors such as abdominal girth, body mass index, fruit and vegetable intake, age, physical activity, taking certain medications and family history (2).

Excess body fat, as measured by body mass index (BMI), and waist circumference are useful measures that reflect various aspects of diet and physical activity and are most strongly associated with the risk of type 2 diabetes mellitus (2).

Waist circumference is useful for measuring visceral fat deposits, and this information is essential when determining risk, due to the mass of fat that can be found accumulated at the peripheral or visceral level. This type of media identifies mainly visceral fat, which contains a large amount of non-esterified fatty acids and produces a higher amount of adipokines, which are associated with increased insulin resistance, thus increasing the risk of DM2 (2).

An important role in the prevention of DM2 is daily physical activity, which increases aerobic capacity and muscle mass, reduces the risk of weight gain and, if performed daily, decreases insulin resistance and thus the risk of developing DM2 (2).

2.8 Chronic Kidney Disease

Chronic kidney disease (CKD), also known as chronic renal failure, is defined as a group of different diseases that affect renal morphology and physiology. The variation in its clinical manifestation is due to aetiopathogenesis, morphological damage (glomerulus, vessels, tubules or renal interstitium), severity and degree of progression (3,12).

The international organisation KDIGO defines CKD as changes in renal structure or function over a period of three months or more, with health consequences regardless of the cause. This means a glomerular filtration rate of less than 60 mL/minute/1.73 m^2, or the occurrence of one or more of the following markers of kidney damage: albuminuria/proteinuria, urine sediment abnormalities, electrolyte abnormalities due to tubular abnormalities, histologically detected abnormalities, structural abnormalities or history of kidney transplantation (Table 3) (3,12).

2.9 Aetiology

Diabetes is the most common cause of kidney disease in the adult population. It is estimated that one third of patients with diabetes develop kidney disease, which is demarcated by albuminuria and/or a decrease in glomerular filtration rate within 15 years after the diagnosis of diabetes has been established (13).

2.10 Epidemiology

It is estimated that in Latin America there are 300 patients with chronic renal failure per million inhabitants, according to the Latin American Society of Nephrology and Hypertension, while the American Academy of Neurology reports that patients with cognitive impairment are investigated from the age of 60 onwards (14).

In Mexico in 2017, the prevalence of CKD was reported to be 12.2% and 51.4 deaths per 100,000 inhabitants. Furthermore, CKD in Mexico has a major impact on the finances of institutions and the economy of families; in 2014, the Ministry of Health estimated annual expenditure for this pathology at 8,966 US dollars (USD), while for the Mexican Social Security Institute it was 9,091 USD (1).

CKD is associated with excessive morbidity, mortality and costs, as well as poor quality of life for patients. In Mexico, the main drawback is particularly serious, as our country ranks first in incidence and sixth in prevalence worldwide. Moreover, the frequency of DM2 is higher in our environment, 12 and this disease is the main cause of ESRD in our country (48% of incident patients on some form of dialysis are diabetic) (14).

2.11 Pathophysiology

When nephron loss occurs, glomerular hypertension induces an increase in nephron size (via activation of the renin-angiotensin system (RAS) and transforming growth factor α (TGFa) and epidermal growth factor receptor (EGFR) activity) as a compensatory mechanism to conserve total GFR and to decrease intraglomerular pressure. As a result, podocytes must undergo hypertrophy to conserve the filtration barrier across the increased filtration surface. In contrast, podocyte hypertrophy is limited, so that beyond a certain threshold, barrier dysfunction first manifests as mild proteinuria when it fails to keep up. In later stages of CKD, increased podocyte shear stress promotes podocyte detachment. Parietal epithelial cells (PECs) are putative podocyte progenitors, but proteinuria and potentially other factors inhibit their potential to replace lost podocytes. However, aggravation causes a response that results in increased scar formation, in the form of focal segmental glomerulosclerosis, global glomerulosclerosis and consequent nephron atrophy. Glomerular hyperfiltration and proteinuria leads to a higher reabsorption workload for the proximal tubules. Subsequently albuminuria, complement and infiltrating immune cells cause tubular cells to secrete proinflammatory mediators that promote interstitial inflammation, along with progression from focal segmental glomerulosclerosis to global glomerulosclerosis promotes tubular atrophy and interstitial fibrosis. Scar formation is associated with vascular rarefaction and ischaemia. As a result, nephron remnants further increase in size to meet filtration demands, accelerating the mechanisms of chronic kidney disease (CKD) progression in a vicious cycle (15).

2.12 Risk factors

Several factors have been identified for the onset and progression of CKD, which may aggravate the primary disease. Several factors have pathophysiological mechanisms in common, such as proteinuria and glomerular hyperfiltration, the most common being and frequent (16).

They are classified into susceptibility factors (which increase the likelihood of kidney damage), initiating factors (those that directly initiate kidney damage), progression factors (which accelerate, worsen and cause more severe functional impairment), and end-stage factors (which contribute to increased morbidity and mortality) (Table 1) (17).

2.12.1 Susceptibility factors (non-modifiable)

Age: not a factor for progression on its own, but due to the deterioration of natural renal function with advancing age. It has been observed that not all patients with advanced age develop an expected decrease in glomerular filtration rate.

Sex: 60% of patients represent the male sex with substitution treatment.

Race: there is a higher incidence in the African-American race, perhaps mostly associated with the prevalence of severe hypertension, socio-cultural status and genetic factors.

Low birth weight: this is associated with a low number of nephrons and the subsequent development of CKD. It is associated with loss of renal mass, in addition to glomerular hypertension or hyperfiltration (16,18).

Socio-cultural deprivation: low social, cultural and economic standards are associated with poorer health, as epidemiological studies show (17).

2.12.2 Susceptibility factors (modifiable)

The factors listed below are indicative of the onset and progression of CKD, but all depend on proteinuria as the main risk factor.

Hypertension: more than 75% of patients suffer from hypertension. Blood pressure below 140/90 mm/Hg is essential in patients with CKD and in patients with diabetes or proteinuria.

Diabetes is one of the most common causes of CKD, occurring in 40-50% of patients. Within which proteinuria is one of the conditioning factors, as well as elevated Hb1ac levels are associated with increased risk.

Obesity: A factor that is most frequently reflected in the general population, overweight is associated with glomerular hyperfiltration.

Dyslipidaemia: has an adverse effect on the vascular system in general. It therefore impacts on the progression of kidney damage.

Smoking: is a cardiovascular factor.

Hyperuricaemia: values higher than 7 mg/dl can lead to uric nephrolithiasis, uric acid nephropathy, tophaceous gout and acute gouty arthritis (16,17,18).

2.12.3 Risk factors capable of directly initiating kidney damage

Autoimmune diseases, systemic infections, urinary tract infections, renal lithiasis, lower urinary tract obstruction, nephrotoxic drugs, mainly NSAIDs, as they are predominantly associated with changes in glomerular haemodynamics.

2.12.4 Risk factors for CKD progression

Proteinuria has a varied mean annual rate of decline in glomerular filtration rate (GFR), from the age of 40 years onwards a normal renal progression rate of 0.7-1 ml/min/1.73 m should be considered[2]. Two measurements of glomerular filtration rate (GFR) and albuminuria levels in three months are recommended, and a decline due to CKD should be excluded (19).

Rapid renal deterioration is related to anaemia and changes in mineral metabolism, particularly hyperphosphataemia. As predictors, it is difficult to isolate the impact of these factors, as they are a consequence of renal damage. However, the early stages of CKD should see correction of anaemia and changes in mineral metabolism (17).

Several studies also identify other risk factors, such as occupational and environmental risks. Chronic exposure to heavy metals such as lead, mercury, cadmium and arsenic can cause severe nephrotoxic effects that can even lead to CKD (20).

Table 3. ERC risk factors

Susceptibility factors: increase the likelihood of kidney damage
Advanced age
Family history of CKD
Decreased renal mass
Low birth weight
Black and other ethnic minorities
Arterial hypertension
Diabetes
Obesity
Low socio-economic status
Initiating factors - directly initiate kidney damage
Autoimmune diseases
Systemic infections
Urinary tract infections
Renal lithiasis
Lower urinary tract obstruction
Nephrotoxic drugs, mainly NSAIDs
Arterial hypertension
Diabetes
Progression factors: worsen renal damage and accelerate renal functional decline
Persistent proteinuria
Poorly controlled high blood pressure
Poorly controlled diabetes
Smoking
Dyslipidaemia
Anemia
Associated cardiovascular disease
Obesity

End-stage factors: increase morbidity and mortality in the setting of renal failure
Low-dose dialysis
Temporary vascular access for dialysis
Anemia
Hypoalbuminaemia
Late referral to nephrology

Source: Levey AS, Stevens LA, Coresh J. Conceptual model of CKD: applications and implications. Am J Kidney Dis. 2009 Mar;53(3 Suppl 3):S4-16.

2.12.5 Diagnosis

Early diagnosis is based on the performance of basic complementary tests to establish the diagnosis and stage of CKD, regardless of the cause (23). There are three basic complementary examinations:

1) Determination of serum creatinine and corresponding estimation of GFR or creatinine clearance using a formula.

2) Determination of the albumin/creatinine ratio in an isolated urine sample.

3) Urine sediment analysis using a urine dipstick or the classical light microscopy technique.

These complementary examinations should be performed in all cases where there is an increased risk of CKD.

According to the clinical practice guidelines for the prevention, diagnosis and treatment of Early Chronic Kidney Disease, renal function should not be assessed by measuring serum creatinine alone, as it is not sufficiently sensitive to provide accurate renal function. Since it can be normal when it is significantly decreased, it is recommended to estimate GFR using the MDRD renal formulas. Alternatively it can be calculated with creatinine clearance using the Cockroft-Gault formula (24).

2.12.6 Classification

According to the KDIGO guidelines classification (table 3), this determines six categories according to GFR and three levels of albuminuria, which suggest the management of the disease, as well as establish the model to be followed within the individualised treatment of the patient during the course of the disease (25).

Table 4. Classification of CKD by GFR* and degree of albuminuria.

				Albuminuria category Description and range		
				A1	A2	A3
				Normal to slightly increased	Moderately increased	Severely increased
				<30 mg/g <3 mg/mmol	30-300 mg/g 3-300 mg/mmol	>300mg/g >30 mg/mmol
GFR* category (ml/min/1.73m) Range and description	GI	Normal high	>90			
	G2	Slightly decreased	60-89			
	G3a	Slightly to moderately decreased	45-59			
	G3b	Moderately to severely impaired	30-44			
	G4	Severely diminished	15-29			
	G5	Renal failure	<15			

Glomerular filtration rate (GFR): Green: Low Risk (if no other markers of kidney disease are present, no CKD. Yellow: Moderately increased risk; Orange: High risk; Red: Very high risk.

Kidney Disease Improving Global Outcomes. KDIGO 2018 Clinical practice guideline for the prevention, diagnosis, evaluation and treatment of hepatitis C in chronic kidney disease. Society of Nephrology 2018; 8(3): 91-165

2.12.7 Treatment

Management of CKD involves reducing albuminuria by treating the underlying causes, mainly diabetes and/or hypertension (22).

Nephroprotection strategies are pharmacological and non-pharmacological measures to limit or prevent the progression of kidney damage, which include: Use of antihypertensives, lipid lowering agents, dietary salt and protein restriction, elimination of tobacco and nephrotoxicants, overweight control (Table 4) (22). Measures are most effective when applied earlier in the course of kidney disease.

Table 5. Non-pharmacological nephroprotective measures.

Non-pharmacological nephroprotective measures	
GFR <60 mg/dL/1.73 m2	Adjust drug dosage according to GFR
	Reducing the risk of AKI due to hypovolemic states
	Prevent AKI due to use of contrast media
	decrease dose or avoid contrast medium
	Consider using isotonic saline solution before, during and after the procedure.
	Defer use of metformin, RAAS blockers and diuretics.
GFR 45 to 60 ml/min/1.73m2	Avoid prolonged use of NSAIDs.
	Continue metformin
GFR 30 - 45 ml/min/173m2	Avoid prolonged use of NSAIDs
	Close monitoring of metformin use at 50% dose.
TFG < 30	Avoid any NSAIDs
	Avoid bisphosphonates
	Avoid metformin
	Use with caution ACE inhibitors and ARBs

Quick Reference Guide. Prevention, Diagnosis and Treatment of Early Chronic Kidney Disease. GPC. Registration Number: IMSS -335-09. ISBN 978-607-8290-04-8

2.13 Prevention

Prevention refers to actions taken to eliminate or minimise the impact of disease and disability. It minimises susceptibility and thus decreases the development of disease, while protecting at-risk groups from aggressive agents to minimise the severity of disease complications (24).

Prevention of CKD risk factors in the population requires systematic educational efforts, such as a balanced diet with trace elements, daily water intake of at least two litres, physical activity, and healthy recreation and non-toxic behaviours (25).

Among the main primary prevention actions are the management of risk factors, such as diabetes mellitus, high blood pressure, etc. These efforts include reducing excessive consumption of saturated fats, smoking, drinking alcohol, taking regular pills or being sedentary for at least eight hours a day, being overweight, obesity, use of nephrotoxic drugs, etc. (25).

2.13.1 Prevention of kidney disease

To prevent progression and complications of CKD, annual proteinuria, microalbuminuria and serum creatinine testing of all patients with a personal pathological history of diabetes mellitus is essential, in addition to specifying personalised and elective measures for each diagnosed patient (25).

If diabetes, proteinuria and low serum bicarbonate are identified as the most important risk factors, the development of chronic kidney disease may be delayed and replacement therapy may be required (26).

High blood pressure and advanced age are also important factors. To determine the causes of kidney disease, it is important to consider the clinical context, such as family and personal history, environmental and social factors, medication use, physical examination, laboratory tests, imaging and pathological diagnoses. Special care is recommended for men and persons with proteinuria, as they are important sources of perpetuating agents of CKD (26).

It is necessary to identify the presence of kidney disease in persons over 50 years of age with hypertension or diabetes, as it is a cost-effective measure in all circumstances. It is suggested to use test strips to determine the amount of albumin in urine and/or to determine the glomerular filtration rate, depending on the availability of these tests (26).

2.13.2 Glycaemic control

The KDIGO and American Diabetes Society (ADA) guidelines state that the most effective intervention to achieve nephroprotection in diabetes mellitus is tight control of glucose levels. Lower haemoglobin A1c values reduce the risk of albuminuria. The risk of developing and progressing to renal disease is mitigated by expected metabolic control. The new anti-diabetic agents iSGLT2 and arGLP1 have been associated with continued prioritisation of metformin therapy (27).

2.13.3 Blood pressure control

Patients with DM2 should aim for blood pressure (BP) levels below 130/80 mmHg to minimise CKD mortality and delay CKD protection, but those with albuminuria may need lower targets due to the potential benefits and risks (27).

To select treatment for hypertension (HTN) in patients with DM2, it involves assessment of albuminuria levels and glomerular filtration rate (GFR) reduction. If GFR is less than 60 ml/min/1.73 mm2 and urinary albumin excretion is greater than 300 mg/g of creatinine, then blocking the renin angiotensin aldosterone system (RAAS) with ACEI or ARAII would be preferred for BP treatment, as it has been shown to prevent progression of CKD (27).

2.13.4 Hygienic - dietary measures

To avoid a sedentary lifestyle, 30 to 60 min of moderate physical activity or exercise 4 to 7 days a week, including moderately vigorous aerobic and/or strength training, and programmes that are tailored to the patient's needs, are suggested (28).

It is recommended to maintain sodium intake at a minimum of 100 mEq/day to maintain sustainable restriction (26).

Diet is a key factor in the prevention and control of kidney disease. A balanced dietary approach that is tailored to the needs of the individual can alleviate many hypertension problems and improve glycaemic control. Three meals per day and 2000 calories per day, including fibre-rich foods, vegetables, reduced amounts of poultry, fish or red meat, reduced sugary drinks, and foods rich in calcium, potassium and magnesium, are recommended to maintain a healthy diet through food (28).

Alcohol consumption above 12-14 g/day, which is equivalent to approximately 300 ml of beer or 150 ml of wine per day, is not recommended, as well as avoiding smoking due to the negative impact on health, such as cardiovascular and renal function (28).

III PROBLEM STATEMENT

The incidence of diabetes mellitus (DM) has been increasing and is now one of the leading causes of death and disability worldwide. In Mexico, 50% of patients with chronic kidney disease are currently secondary to DM (23).

CKD represents a catastrophic public health problem due to the high cost and high morbidity and mortality or disability requiring treatment for patients. As a consequence of the new lifestyle, it has led to an increase in the prevalence and incidence of chronic degenerative diseases, particularly DM and systemic arterial hypertension (23).

It is important that people with type 2 diabetes have adequate glycaemic control at the time of diagnosis and are aware of and take appropriate preventive measures in their daily lives to avoid CKD.

In this sense, our role as physicians is to provide patients with the necessary information to prevent complications and delay renal function by identifying potential risk factors. This allows us to prolong renal replacement therapy.

Hence the importance of the present study for which the following research question is posed:

Research question

What are the risk factors for the onset and progression of CKD in patients with DM2 at UMF No 49?

IV JUSTIFICATION

MAGNITUDE: CKD currently has an increasing prevalence and incidence, mainly due to the presence of previous pathologies such as diabetes and mainly affecting the most socially disadvantaged population. Early identification of risk factors can lead to early intervention to prevent kidney damage.

TRANSCENDENCE: is of utmost relevance, as early identification of risk factors for CKD in patients with DM2 could reduce the possible complications derived from the disease and intervene early in the prevention of kidney damage.

IMPACT: the results obtained could be considered as an area of opportunity to propose or carry out improvements in care, to implement programmes and strategies to delay the progression of CKD in this group of patients, reducing the epidemiological and economic impact.

FEASIBILITY: this study was possible to identify predisposing factors to CKD in the population with DM2 in the UMF No. 49 to be studied, it was easy to carry out during the family medicine consultation, and the resources invested did not involve a large cost.

V HYPOTHESIS

It was decided to dispense with hypotheses because of the type of study design.

VI OBJECTIVES

III.1 General Objective

To identify risk factors for the onset and progression of CKD in patients with DM2 at UMF No 49.

III.2 Specific Objectives

1. Quantify and describe the risk factors in the study population.
2. Identify the most frequent susceptibility factor.
3. To determine the most frequent factor of progression in patients with type 2 diabetes.
4. Describo the frequency of susceptibility factors, onset and progression according to age and gender.

VII MATERIALS AND METHODS

III.3 Place

Family Medicine Unit No. 49, IMSS, Durango, Durango

III.4 Universe

Patients with Type 2 Diabetes at Family Medicine Unit No 49

III.5 Weather

The implementation period will be from January to February 2024.

III.6 Study design

It is an observational, descriptive, retrospective study.

III.7 Selection criteria

7.5.1 Inclusion criteria:

1. Patient files of patients over 18 years of age
2. Patient records of either sex.
3. Patient records of patients with a diagnosis of type 2 diabetes mellitus assigned to UMF 49.

7.5.2 Exclusion criteria:

1. Records of patients undergoing renal replacement therapy.
2. Files with insufficient information.
3. File not available.
4. Patients with chronic kidney disease in KDIGO stages 3a, 3b and 4.

III.8 Sample size and sampling

It was calculated with the EPIDAT programme using as an assumption the interactive map of the distribution of the IMSS beneficiary population of the Family Medicine Unit No. 49 (UMF 49) reporting a total of 108, 561 (65); as an expected proportion we used the press release no. 645/21 (66) which reports a prevalence of diabetes of

10.32%; a confidence level of 95% and an absolute precision of 5%; resulting in a total of 139 files.

III.9 Study variables

Variable name	Conceptual definition	Operational definition	Type of variable	Scale	Categories or units of measurement
Age	A person's lifespan from birth to a certain point in time.	Years referred to in the file .	Quantitative Continua	Reason.	Number of years
Sex	The condition of an organism that distinguishes between male and female.	Organic status referred to in the dossier	Qualitative Dichotomous	Nominal.	1. Male 2. Female
Nutritional status	A person's nutrient status in relation to the nutrients in his or her diet.	Categories based on the Body Mass Index (kg/m2) recorded in the file: a. <18.5 = Underweight b. 8.5-24.9 = Normal c. 25-29.9 = Overweight d. >30 = Obesity	Qualitative Ordinal	Ordinal	1. Underweight 2. Normal 3. Overweight 4. Obesity
Body weight	The amount of mass that a person's body holds.	Weight recorded in the electronic medical record.	Continuous quantitative.	Reason	Kilograms
Size	Height of a person, measured from the sole of the foot to the vertex of the head.	Height recorded in the electronic health record.	Continuous quantitative.	Reason	Metres
Susceptibility factors in CKD	State of being predisposed or susceptible to developing the possibility of kidney damage	Factors recorded or described in the dossier: 1. Advanced age (over 60 years) 2. Family history of CKD 3. Arterial hypertension 4. Diabetes	Qualitative Polytomous	Nomination	1. Yes 2. No

		5. Obesity			
Initiating factors for CKD	They are those that can directly initiate kidney damage.	Factors recorded or described in the dossier: 1 Autoimmune diseases (rheumatological pathology Systemic Lupus Erythematosus and Rheumatoid Arthritis). 2 Renal Lithiasis 3 Nephrotoxic drugs (NSAIDS)	Qualitative Polytomous	Nominal	1. Yes 2. No
Factors in the progression of CKD	Any event capable of worsening pre-existing glomerular damage.	Factors recorded or described in the dossier: 1.Poorly controlled hypertension (BP >130/80 mm Hg) 2.Poorly controlled diabetes (fasting glucose >130 mg/dl or HbA1C > 7%)3. Smoking 4. Dyslipidaemia 5. Anaemia	Qualitative Polytomous	Nomination	1. Yes 2. No

III.10 Study procedure

7.8.1 Phase I. Authorisations.

With prior authorisation from the Local Research Committee (CLIS 902), and the Local Research Ethics Committee (CEI 9028), based at UMF No. 43 in Gómez Palacio, Durango, also in accordance with the authorisation of the director of family medicine unit No. 49 by means of a letter of no inconvenience.

7.8.2 Phase II. Method of selection of subjects or study units.

With prior authorisation, the case selection process will begin, reviewing the clinical records of type 2 Diabetes Mellitus patients from UMF 49 Durango at for a period from January 2024 to February 2024.

7.8.3 Phase III. Data collection.

Data will be collected from patient records through the family medicine information system (SIMF) and will be captured on a data collection sheet, which is found in the appendix, a folio will be assigned to each subject, the presence of risk factors will be recorded, which will be classified by susceptibility factors (modifiable and non-modifiable), initiation factors and progression factors for chronic kidney disease recorded in the clinical records of patients with type 2 Diabetes Mellitus of the different shifts of care of the UMF 49.

7.8.4 Phase IV. Information management.

The information obtained through the data collection sheet will be captured in an Excel database, for subsequent statistical analysis using SPSS V25 software. It will be kept confidential, as well as ensuring that it will not be used for anything other than scientific and dissemination purposes.

III.11 Statistical analysis

To determine the research objectives, a descriptive statistical approach will be used. For qualitative variables (sex), frequencies and percentages will be used; for quantitative variables (age), measures of central tendency (median, mean) and measures of dispersion (standard deviations, minimum and maximum) will be used. Quantitative variables with normal distribution will be described with the mean accompanied by the standard deviation; while quantitative variables with non-normal distribution will be described with the median, accompanied by minima and maxima. Statistical significance will be estimated considering a confidence interval of 95% or a p-value <0.05. The information for each variable will be entered into a database Microsoft Excel programme, using the statistical package SPSS version 25 for Windows, to subsequently analyse the results obtained in order to draw conclusions and make recommendations.

VIII RESULTS AND DISCUSSION

Table 6 shows the percentage frequency of men and women with diabetes mellitus, of which in the total sample (139) the female population with diabetes mellitus was 28% higher than the percentage of men. These results are different from those found by Fernández and Melgosa (2022), who reported that CKD was more frequent in males, which is caused by the renal damage produced by DM2.

Table 6. Frequency of sex of the auscultated sample with DM2 in the UMF No. 49 in Ciudad Victoria Durango, Durango.

SEX	*FREQUENCY*	*PERCENTAGE*
Male	*50*	36%
Female	89	64%
Total	139	100%

SUSCEPTIBILITY FACTORS:

The frequency of nutritional status considering the weight of patients with DM2 can be seen in Table 7, from which it could be estimated that the highest percentage corresponded to patients with obesity, who were 46.8, 27.4 and 15.8% higher than those who were underweight, normal weight or overweight. The mean weight was 76.4 kg, in a sample with a normal distribution and a standard deviation (σ) of 16.2 kg with respect to the above-mentioned mean. The mean height was 1.6, σ=0.09, with normal distribution. These results are also related to those published by Riddle (2019), since this author mentions that abdominal perimeter (obesity) and body mass index are risk factors that contribute to generate conditions for susceptibility to DM2 and CKD.

Frequency of nutritional status according to weight in patients with DM2 in UMF No. 49 in Ciudad Victoria Durango, Durango.

NUTRITIONAL STATUS	*FRACUENCY*	*PERCENTAGE*
Low weight	1	0.7%
Normal	28	20.1%
Overweight	44	31.7%
Obesity	66	47.5%
Total	139	100%

The number of records reviewed belonging to patients over 60 years of age with DM2 and at risk of CKD can be seen in table 8, so that of the total sample (139) it was found that the majority of patients did have DM2 and CKD, which was 12.2% higher than the group of patients who did not have DM2 and CKD. Statistical analyses indicated that the sample had a normal distribution, with a mean of 59.4 and standard deviation=13.0 (absolute deviation from the mean). These results indicate that age, as a risk factor for developing DM2 and, consequently, CKD, is related to that mentioned by Riddle (2019) on age as a risk factor for DM2, as well as to that reported by Zamora and Sanahuja (2008) and López *et al.* (2020), who refer that the age of individuals with glomerular flow (GFR) deficiency or outside normal is a factor that leads to the development of CKD.

Frequency of age >60 years in patients with DM2 in UMF No. 49 in Ciudad Victoria Durango, Durango.

>60 YEARS	***FREQUENCY***	**PERCENTAGE**
Yes	78	56.1%
No	61	43.9%
Total	139	100%

This research conducted on patients with DM2 and arterial hypertension (AHT) showed that the latter risk factor for developing CKD was 48.2% more frequent in the part of the sample of patients with AHT (103) compared to the number of people (36) who had not yet developed CKD (Table 9). The aforementioned results are in line with Mejía *et al.* (2018) that HTN is a risk factor for kidney damage that often appears in patients with DM2. Likewise, with those of García-Maset *et al.* (2021), who have pointed out that kidney damage or CKD is related to HTN, which when undetected and not treated in a timely manner can occur more frequently in the population with DM2.

Table 9. Frequency of arterial hypertension in patients with DM2 in UMF No. 49 of Ciudad Victoria Durango, Durango.

HIGH BLOOD PRESSURE	FREQUENCY	*PERCENTAGE*
Yes	103	74.1%
No	36	25.9%
Total	139	100%

INITIATING FACTORS:

Table 10 contains the results on the frequency of autoimmune diseases in patients with DM2 in UMF No. 49 in Ciudad Victoria Durango, Durango. 49 in Ciudad Victoria Durango, Durango, which showed that of the total sample, the group of patients who did not yet have this type of problem was 87% higher than the group that had developed this type of disease, which suggested continuing with diagnosis and prevention in those patients who do not yet have it, to delay renal damage with serious consequences that can lead to CKD; however, these results also indicated not to neglect the few who have already developed it and, as far as possible, delay the stage of greatest renal deterioration in patients.

Frequency of autoimmune diseases in patients with DM2 in UMF No. 49 in Ciudad Victoria Durango, Durango.

AUTOIMMUNE DISEASES	*FREQUENCY*	*PERCENTAGE*
Yes	9	6.5%
No	130	93.5%
Total	139	100%

The frequency of nephrotoxic drugs in the total sample (139) of patients, corresponding to UMF No. 49 in Ciudad Victoria Durango, Durango, is indicated by the absolute values and percentages in Table 11, from which it was possible to estimate that nephrotoxic drugs have not yet been developed in most of the sample of patients, which in turn exceeded by 12.2% the number of patients who have already developed this problem.

Frequency of nephrotoxic drugs in patients with DM2 in UMF No. 49 in Ciudad Victoria Durango, Durango.

NEPHROTOXIC DRUGS	FREQUENCY	PERCENTAGE
Yes	61	43.9%
No	78	56.1%
Total	139	100%

PROGRESSION FACTORS:

The results regarding the risk factor for CKD, known as frequency of poorly controlled arterial hypertension, are shown in Table 12, with which it was detected that this risk factor did occur in UMF No. 49 in Ciudad Victoria Durango, Durango, although it should be noted that it was only detected in the smallest part of the total sample (139 patients with DM2) reviewed through the respective files. 49 of Ciudad Victoria Durango, Durango, although it should be noted that it was only detected in the smallest part of the total sample (139) of patients with DM2 reviewed through the respective files; also, that in most of the sample population the same deficiency in control of arterial hypertension has not occurred, so it was possible to estimate that the frequency of poorly controlled arterial hypertension was exceeded by 64% by the number of patients without the aforementioned problem. This also suggests that it is necessary to reduce the number of cases with the problem in question and thus avoid, as far as possible, the recurrence of this factor in the progression of arterial hypertension.

Table 12. Frequency of poorly controlled hypertension (BP >130/80mm/Hg).

HIGH BLOOD PRESSURE POORLY CONTROLLED	*FREQUENCY*	*PERCENTAGE*
Yes	*25*	18%
No	*114*	82%
Total	139	100%

Table 13 contains the results on the frequency of poorly controlled diabetes, which showed that the number of cases with this risk factor for the progression of DM2 and consequently CKD was 9.4% less compared to the number of cases without the problem that has consequences for the progression of both diseases. However, these results also suggest that it is necessary to reduce the problem in question so that it does not overtake the number of cases without the problem, and so that it does not become one of the main risk factors in the two diseases suffered by patients at UMF No. 49 in Ciudad Victoria Durango, Durango.

Table 13. Frequency of poorly controlled diabetes (fasting glucose >130mg/dl or hbac1 >7%).

POORLY CONTROLLED DIABETES	*FREQUENCY*	*PERCENTAGE*

Yes	*63*	*45.3%*
No	*76*	54.7%
Total	139	100%

The review of records of patients with DM2 in FMU No. 49 also revealed that smoking is another problem faced by some IMSS beneficiaries in the aforementioned FMU, but occurs less frequently, as indicated by the results in Table 14, which clearly shows that the percentage of patients with smoking problems reported in the respective records is 75.6% higher than in the group of patients who do not use tobacco; however, it is still important to continue with activities that lead patients to distance themselves from this risk factor for DM2 and CKD.6% by the group of patients who do not use tobacco; nevertheless, it is still important to continue with activities that lead patients to distance themselves from this risk factor for DM2 and CKD, since according to the Clinical Practice Guideline (2014) smoking is a risk and progression factor that is associated with reduced renal function.

Table 14. Frequency of smoking in patients with DM2 in UMF No. 49 in Ciudad Victoria Durango, Durango.

TOBACISM	*FREQUENCY*	*PERCENTAGE*
Yes	17	12.2%
No	122	87.8%
Total	139	100%

Dyslipidaemia is another risk factor for the progression of DM2 and CKD that was found in the records of patients at UMF No.49 in Ciudad Victoria Durango, Durango. of Ciudad Victoria Durango, Durango, which consists of an elevated concentration of cholesterol and/or triglycerides or a low concentration of high-density lipoprotein (HDL) cholesterol , the results of which can be seen in Table 15, which in turn indicated that this factor affected patients less frequently and in a lower percentage, such that the group without dyslipidaemia was 41% higher than the group with dyslipidaemia; However, the results also suggest that this factor needs to be addressed in patients who have already developed dyslipidaemia, before the number of patients with the problem increases and it is considered a risk factor with increasing frequency.

Table 15. Frequency of dyslipidaemia in patients with DM2 in UMF No. 49 in Ciudad Victoria Durango, Durango.

DYSLIPIDEMIA	*FREQUENCY*	*PERCENTAGE*
Yes	*41*	29.5%
No	98	70.5%
Total	139	100%

Anaemia is a problem that occurs as a result of low numbers of functional (healthy) red blood cells, or because there is not enough haemoglobin to transport oxygen to the other cells, tissues and organs of the person. Table 16 reports the results found through the respective records of patients with DM2 in the UMF No. 49 of the IMSS in Ciudad Victoria Durango, Durango, results which indicated that anaemia is a factor with a low frequency in the aforementioned patients, to such an extent that it was exceeded by 94.2% by the group of people who do not have anaemia. Even with this low frequency of anaemia, it is important to do what is necessary to further reduce or eliminate the frequency of the disease in question.

Table 16. Frequency of patients with anaemia and DM2 in UMF No. 49 in Ciudad Victoria Durango, Durango.

ANEMIA	*FREQUENCY*	*PERCENTAGE*
Yes	*4*	2.9%
No	135	97.1%
Total	139	100%

IX CONCLUSIONS

This research showed that the main risk factors for the onset and progression of CKD in patients with DM2 in the UMF No. 49 of the IMSS in Ciudad Victoria Durango, Durango, were gender, nutritional status, age, high blood pressure, poorly controlled diabetes and nephrotoxic drugs; while factors such as autoimmune diseases, poorly controlled high blood pressure, smoking, dyslipidaemia and anaemia were not very frequent in the population used for the research. However, they also require attention to reduce them further in the population with DM2 and CKD treated at UMF No. 49. These results also apply to all those with DM2 and CKD in the country and elsewhere in the world.

X PERSPECTIVES

The results of this research can be applied to increase the quality of the medical service offered at the UMF No. 49 of the IMSS in Ciudad Victoria Durango, Durango, to care for patients with DM2 and at risk of developing CKD. This can only be achieved by improving the knowledge of medical and auxiliary staff to increase their effectiveness in the treatment of DM2 and CKD suffered by patients at UMF No. 49. Also, to increase the effectiveness of medical and auxiliary staff in the application of knowledge to prevent the onset and progression of DM2 and CKD, by improving knowledge to detect major and minor risk factors.

On the other hand, with this knowledge generated through research, it will be possible to improve information on CKD, and perhaps participate more effectively in the transmission of knowledge to medical, auxiliary and other personnel in IMSS institutions in the state of Durango and at national level, as well as in other public (Ministry of Health) or private institutions, also at state and national level. In turn, the UMF No. 49 of the IMSS in Ciudad Victoria Durango, Durango, will be able to influence national development in terms of the health of citizens who have developed CKD. Furthermore, with the results generated so far, the possibilities of contributing knowledge to health science in general, specifically on the subject of kidney damage, will increase if the information is organised in the form of a scientific article for publication in a scientific journal, or a book chapter with editorial authorisation. If this is done, it will increase the possibilities of influencing the internationalisation of the knowledge generated in UMF No. 49 and, therefore, of the institution itself and of the staff responsible for the publication.

XI BIBLIOGRAPHICAL REFERENCES

1. Obrador GT, Rubilar X, Agazzi E, Estefan J. The Challenge of Providing Renal Replacement Therapy in Developing Countries: The Latin American Perspective. American journal of kidney diseases: the official journal of the National Kidney Foundation. 2016. Mar;67(3):499-506. Available in: https://doi.org/10.1053/j.ajkd.2015.08.033

2. Riddle MC. STANDARDS OF MEDICAL CARE IN DIABETES. American Diabetes Association [Internet]. 2019;42. Available from: https://care.diabetesjournals.org/content/diacare/suppl/2018/12/17/42.Supplement_1.DC1/DC_42_S1_2019_UPDATED.pdf

3. García-Maset R, et al. Information and consensus document for the detection and management of chronic kidney disease. Nefrología. 2021. https://doi.org/10.1016/j.nefro.2021.07.010

4. Del M, Mejía Gómez C, González Espíndola A, Mendoza IL, Cervantes SL, Carlos J, et al. Articles published in this journal are distributed under the license: Articles [Internet]. Available from: http://dx.doi.org/10.19230/jonnpr.2625

5. Ángel, M., Valdés, S., Serra, M., Marleny, R., & García, V. (2019). Noncommunicable chronic diseases: current magnitude and future trends Non Transmissible Chronic Diseases : Current Magnitude and. 5-11. Retrieved from http://www.revfinlay.sld.cu/index.php/finlay/article/view/561/1658

6. Overview of diabetes in the Region of the Americas [Internet]. Pan American Health Organization; 2023 [cited 2024 Jan 9]. Available from: https://iris.paho.org/handle/10665.2/57197

7. The Standards of Medical Care in Diabetes 2021, redGDPS summary (ADA 2021) [Internet]. Redgdps.org [cited 2024 Jan 9]. Available from: https://www.redgdps.org/los-standards-of-medical-care-in-diabetes-2021- summary-

redgdps-ada-2021

8. Porto J, Gardey A. Definition of knowledge [cited 07 Nov 2021]. Available from: https://www.significados.com/conocimiento/

9. IDF (2017). IDF Diabetes Atlas. In International Diabetes Federation (Octava). https://doi.org/10.1016/j.diabres.2017.09.002

10. Colagiuri ARW. IDF DIABETES ATLAS. copyright; 2019.

11. Garmendia-Lorena F. El tratamiento actual de la Diabetes Mellitus tipo 2. diagnostico (lima) [Internet]. 2020; Available from: http://doi.org/10.33734/diagnostico.v59i1.200G

12. Ammirati AL. Chronic kidney disease. Rev Assoc Med Bras [Internet]. 2020;66(suppl 1):s03-9. Available from: http://dx.doi.org/10.1590/1806-9282.66.s1.3

13. Alicic RZ, Rooney MT, Tuttle KR. Diabetic kidney disease: challenges, progress, and possibilities. Clin J Am Soc Nephrol. 2017 Dec 7;12(12):2032-45.(https://cjasn.asnjournals.org/content/12/12/2032)

14. Gómez-Andrade LF, Lindao-Solano MO. Association between Non-Terminal Chronic Kidney Disease and Cognitive Impairment in Adults aged 55-65 years. Ecuadorian Journal of Neurology. 2020;29.

15. Rui Sheng Cen Feng, Karina Hernández Gonza, Shaylinn Mena Sánchez, Daniela Zamora Chaves, Jeremy Zeledón López. Chronic Kidney Disease. Clinical Journal of the UCR-HSJD School of Medicine [Internet]. 2020;10. Available from: https://www.medigraphic.com/pdfs/revcliescmed/ucr-2020/ucr204i.pdf

16. Sanahuja IZ and MJ. Enfermedad renal crónica. Asoc. Española Pediatría 2008;9: 110.

17. Lorenzo Sellarés V, Luis Rodríguez D. Chronic Kidney Disease. in: Lorenzo V., López Gómez JM (Eds). Nefrología al día. ISSN: 2659-2606. Available at:

https://www.nefrologiaaldia.org/136

18. López-Heydeck S. M, Robles-Navarro J. B, Montenegro-Morales L. P, Garduño-García J. D, López-Arriaga J. A. Risk and lifestyle factors associated with chronic kidney disease. Revista Médica del Instituto Mexicano del Seguro Social [Internet]. 2020;58(3):305-316. Retrieved from: https://www.redalyc.org/articulo.oa?id=457768136013

19. Martínez-Castelao Alberto, Górriz José L., Bover Jordi, Segura-de la Morena Julián, Cebollada Jesús, Escalada Javier et al . Consensus document for the detection and management of chronic kidney disease. Nefrología (Madr.) [Internet]. 2014 [cited 2024 Jan 16] ; 34(2): 243-262. Available from: http://scielo.isciii.es/scielo.php?script=sci arttext&pid=S0211- 69952014000200014 &lng=en.ttps://dx.doi.org/10.3265/Nefrologia.pre2014.Feb.12455.

20. Ana María Iraizoz Barrios, Germán Brito Sosa, Jovanny Angelina Santos Luna. Detection of risk factors for chronic kidney disease in adults. Cuban Journal of General Comprehensive Medicine. 2022;38(2):1745.

21. Cabrera SS. Definition and classification of the stages of chronic kidney disease. Prevalence. Keys to early diagnosis. Risk factors for chronic kidney disease. Nefrología. Vol 24. Supplement No. 6 Chapter 2 2016;27-34

22. Quick Reference Guide. Prevention, Diagnosis and Treatment of Early Chronic Kidney Disease. GPC. Registration Number: IMSS -33509. ISBN 978-607-8290-04-8

23. Gómez LDO. Chronic kidney disease and survival factors in kidney transplant patients. Rev Salud y Bienestar Social, Vol 5. 1 January-June 2021;

24. Lizbeth Estefanía Cárdenas Suárez, Gabriela Alexandra Carpio Vaca, Jessica Ximena Humala Rojas, Lesly Marcela Verdugo Calle. Chapter II. Health promotion and prevention in society. Public Health CON-CIENCIAISBN; 2022.

25. Núñez-López M, Triana-Alonso P, Licea-Morales Y. Application of levels of

prevention in chronic kidney disease. Revista Finlay [journal on the Internet]. 2018 [cited 2018 Oct 22]; 8(3): [approx. 1 p.]. Available from: http://revfinlay.sld.cu/index.php/finlay/article/view/614

26. Prevention, Diagnosis and Treatment of Chronic Kidney Disease. Guía de Evidencias y Recomendaciones: Guía de Práctica Clínica. Mexico, CENETEC; 2019 [9 January 2024]. Available at: http://imss.gob.mx/profesionales- salud/gpc

27. Beatriz Fernández Fernández AO. Treatment of diabetic kidney disease. Nefrología al Día [Internet]. 2021 May 13; Available from: https://www.nefrologiaaldia.org/es-articulo-tratamiento-enfermedad-renal- diabetica-394

28. García-Maset R, Bover J, Segura de la Morena J, Goicoechea Diezhandino M, Cebollada del Hoyo J, Escalada San Martín J, et al. Information and consensus document for the detection and management of chronic kidney disease. Nefrología. [Internet]. 2022;42(3):233-64. Available from: https://www.sciencedirect.com/science/article/pii/S0211699521001612

29. PDA | Tableau Public [Internet]. [cited 2022 Aug 4]. Available from: https://public.tableau.com/app/profile/imss.cpe/viz/PDA/DSH PDA

30. STATISTICS ON WORLD DIABETES DAY (14 NOVEMBER) NATIONAL DATA [cited 2022 Aug 4]; Available from: https://www.paho.org/es/campanas/dia-mundial-diabetes-2020

31. Fernández C. C. and Marta Melgosa H. M. 2022. Chronic kidney disease (CKD) in childhood: diagnosis and treatment. Protoc diagn ter pediatr 1:437-457.

32. Mejía, G. M. del C., Alejandro Gónzalez E. A., Israel López M. I, Latorre C. S. and Ruvalcaba L. J. C. 2018. Risk factors for kidney damage in patients with type 2 diabetes in the first level of care. Journal of Negative and No Positive Result 3(10): 825-837.

33. Clinical Practice Guideline. 2014. Treatment of type 2 diabetes mellitus in the first level of care, Mexico. Mexico: Instituto Mexicano del Seguro Social. https://www.gob.mx/salud/cenetec.

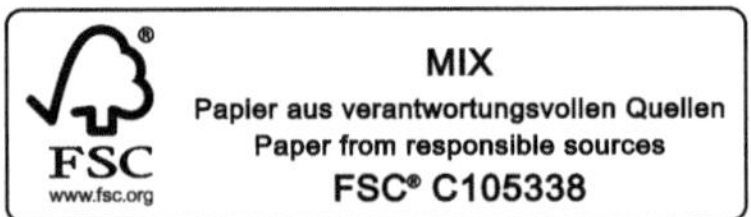

Printed by Books on Demand GmbH, Norderstedt / Germany